Question:

What is the one thing you could do, such that by doing it everything else will be easier or unnecessary?

www.thestress-lesslife.com

First published in 2016

1

Text copyright © Michael Adu, 2016

My Why...

The reason I started off my business and wrote this book is because I feel like the world's health is in decline. We, as a community, are heading to premature death and illness. I don't feel that this is the way we were supposed to live and I don't feel like this is the way we are supposed to be.

My pursuit for knowledge in the arenas of holistic health and stress management is very personal to me, and I am very passionate about this subject. This is mainly because it rings closely to my personal life and my personal relationships.

I have personally been through mental health issues, namely anxiety. It started for me when I was a teenager. I didn't feel like a normal teenager because, in certain situations, I would overreact, sometimes hyperventilate, and on the rare occasion, physically be sick. I knew this behaviour wasn't normal as I analysed my own behaviour and characteristics with other peoples' characteristics. Why did my body react in this way?

As I got older, I felt like I had no-one to speak to. It felt like no-one knew what I was going through.

I started to do research on the mind and the psychology of emotions, feelings and thoughts. I've researched people like Carol Dweck, Tony Robbins, Deepak Chopra, Paul Chek and other inspirational leaders in the field of self-development, mental mastery and the pursuit of holistic health. I began to work on myself, from the inside out. From learning about breathing techniques, exercise and energy building activities, meditation, the healing powers of food, hormone balancing, emotional intelligence, metacognition, mind-set training and mastery, cold pressed juices and postural assessment and massage, I have developed my own holistic health and stress management programmes for individuals and corporations. I feel like the only way to obtain a true sense of health is to look at you as a living organism. Your body is reproducing 10 million cells per second, and everything that you do is affecting whether the cells are going to be healthy and strong, or diminish in strength. We are in full control of our bodies, our states, our minds and what we eat. We need to take back the power from health professionals and let it remain in our own hands.

All aspects of health are 100% connected. One aspect of health affects another so if you want to be physically strong, mental strength has to come into play. It is not one or the other. This is the philosophy of living this Stress-Less way of life. Working on you as a whole.

The other reason I set up this business is because of the health risks exposed to the general public. Hard-working citizens who are working sometimes 40+ hours per week have no service that helps them obtain a true sense of health. This is the case with some of my immediate family members who have contracted illnesses and diseases through hard-working and dedication to the job with no regard to health. This, coupled with a poor diet and exercise routine, is a recipe for disaster.

When my father contracted two forms of cancer, the message really hit home. He dedicated his life to working hard and building a home for himself and his family. Questioning him on how he feels, he said that he hasn't felt healthy or pain-free in the last two years. He is now taking medication to control this illness. This is the sad reality for a lot of individuals who live in the western world.

I made a commitment to myself and to my family that I would create this business and help people move towards a more wellness focused lifestyle. A life where small changes create massive results. A life of no pain, vitality and happiness.

Using the philosophy of my company, Stress-Less, I have delivered programmes for my father and for many others in the pursuit of holistic health.

Come and experience the Stress-Less Way of life.

Contents

Current situation

We are living in a society where health issues are increasing rapidly. In the 1980's, the rate of an individual being diagnosed with cancer was one in every 8 people. In our current environment, it is 1 in 2 people born after 1960.

Cancer Research UK, http://www.cancerresearchuk.org/health-professional/cancer-statistics/risk/lifetime-risk#heading-Zero, Accessed Nov 2015

New diseases are appearing that were not contracted 100 years ago. Our current efforts to increase health and vitality are non-effective at best. Trillions have been injected into medical research. There has been some advancement in the field of medicine, yet we are a community of human beings that are dying faster than ever.

Our current model of health is disease focused wellness, meaning once an individual is diagnosed with a disease or ailment, they are prescribed medication to counteract the symptoms with the intention of making the individual feel better.

This model of disease based wellness has some major flaws attached.

Firstly, it is focused on fixing the symptoms and not the cause of the symptoms. For example, if I have a headache, I take paracetamol to take away the pain. It doesn't tackle the root cause of a headache. Our body is a sophisticated and intelligent organism that does not exhibit pain for no particular reason, it is trying to alert you that something is not right and something needs to change to bring you back to a state of health. If we are just taking away the symptoms without addressing the root cause of the problem, our body will keep trying to initiate change with no prevail, creating illnesses and dis-ease.

Secondly, when we rely solely on medication for health, this gives one industry in particular sole rights to benefits from this model, pharmaceutical companies. I am not slating pharmaceutical companies, many of them have done great work in advancement to medical science. I am only stating that when we rely on one industry to treat and heal us, there may be some within the industry that may not want to see another form of health or healing come into the frame for financial reasons.

Thirdly, we have no control of our own health. We go on living blind to what our diet, our activity levels, thoughts, feelings, quality of the air we breathe in, energy that surrounds us and the energy that modern science inflicts on us; is doing to us and our physiology. There has been a massive increase of the amount of foreign agents attacking our system. These agents are relatively new and our body doesn't know how to deal with them. These create imbalances in the body creating dis-ease and illness.

We need to move towards a new way of thinking, a new way of looking at health. The Stress-Less Way of Life. This way is a new wellness approach where we work on a 'prevention before cure' model. We take ownership of our own health, our minds, our body and our life.

Wellness focused health is about making relatively minor changes to your lifestyle and in return, you will feel better and decrease the chances of contracting an illness or dis-ease.

By doing this, you can increase the longevity and vitality in your life.

Start now and live the Stress-Less Life.

Current state- Physical

Current facts:

- *21% of young men and 16% of young women meet the recommended exercise guidelines of an hour a day.*

- *Individuals on a low-income exercise less than those on a high income – 21% less in men and 16% in women*

- *There is a clear association between meeting the UK exercise guidelines and being overweight or obese.*

Health and Social Care Information Centre. http://www.hscic.gov.uk/catalogue/PUB13648/Obes-phys-acti-diet-eng-2014-rep.pdf, Accessed on March 2015

Current activity levels of individuals in the UK:

The true art of effective movement is lost. Those who are moving, in relation to the people who are predominantly static, are promoting poor posture and causing changes in their body composition. Tight hamstrings, inactive Gluteus Maximus (derrière), body curvature and hunched over shoulders are all results of lack of or poor movement. There is also a large portion of people who are not moving enough on a day to day basis. With the muscle we attribute to movement, it is the case that if you don't use it, you lose it.

Muscles can start to decrease by a rate of 1% in your 30's, increasing the chances of injuries. This condition is called sarcopenia with aging. Also, your heart becomes less accustomed to stress if unexercised. Stress for the heart caused by exercise can be beneficial as it gives the heart a chance to become a lot more effective in its mission to supply your body with oxygen and energy. This in turn can reduce blood pressure, improve circulation and have multiple health benefits.

For those who exercise and are trying to develop healthy habits through exercise, I applaud you. One issue that is rarely addressed with exercisers is over-exercising and over-stressing.

Over-exercising is a term describing an individual exercising intensively and not giving their body enough time to rebuild and grow from exercise. The purpose of exercise is for our body to grow and become stronger. In order for this to happen, we need to give our body adequate rest to rebuild. The two main processes of cells are categorised as anabolic and catabolic reactions.

Anabolism is the process in the body which focuses on regeneration and growth. It is when the body is in optimal digestion and everything is moving in optimal synchronicity for repair. Hormones associated with repair e.g. serotonin, are released at this time.

Catabolism is the process in the body associated with stress. Fight or flight symptoms are turned on e.g. heart rate increases, pupils dilate, adrenaline and cortisol are released etc. When this happens, all energy is taken away from digestion and other non-vital functions. The primary objective is to survive the stressful state.

Now, if your body is being constantly stressed through exercise, it doesn't have enough time to become effectively anabolic and grow/learn from previous stresses.

Over-stressing is very similar to over-exercising. It is a state when your body becomes too stressed. The only difference is that the stress does not have to be from exercise. Having an intensive work lifestyle which only allows you little to no downtime and in a constant state of stress is a form of being over-stressed. Repetitive strain injury is a form of over-stress on the physical body. There are many forms of over stressing of the body. It can affect people in different ways as we experience stress differently and it manifests in different forms.

Current state- Mental

Current facts:

- **One in four this year will develop some sort of mental health issue**

- **One in ten children are registered with mental health issues**

Mental Health Foundation. Retrieved from
http://www.mentalhealth.org.uk/help-information/mental-health-statistics/
Accessed on Nov 2015.

- **Stress, depression and anxiety cost 9.9 million sick days in 2014/2015.**

Health and Safety Executive. Retrieved from
http://www.hse.gov.uk/statistics/causdis/stress/ Accessed on Nov 2015

- **20% of UK students feel likely to have a mental condition and 13% of students have suicidal thoughts during stressful periods**

National University Service. Retrieved from http://www.nus.org.uk/en/news/20-
per-cent-of-students-consider-themselves-to-have-a-mental-health-problem/.
Accessed in Nov 2015

An area of health that is becoming more prominent now is mental health. It was overlooked in the past, but it is now one of the world's most up and coming problems with the World Health Organisation indicating that by 2020, depression could be one of the biggest problems in the world.

World Health Organisation. Retrieved from
http://www.who.int/mental_health/advocacy/en/Call_for_Action_MoH_Intro.pdf
. Accessed on Nov 2015

As stress is so subjective and it is different for everyone, it can be hard to measure and hard to treat. Each person interprets day-to-day stress in different ways. Therefore, they have adopted an approach of waiting for symptoms of mental health and then treating it from medication and psychotherapy.

<u>Depression</u>

Let's start off by looking at depression. Everyone has ups and downs, everyone has low times and grief from losing a loved one. It is common for people to say they feel depressed at this time, but it doesn't mean that they are in depression.

Depression is a mood disorder characterised by a low mood and the wide range of other possible symptoms, which varies from person to person. This illness can be developed quickly or gradually, and can be brought on by life events and/or changes in the body's chemistry.

It is a common mental illness that is recognised worldwide, affecting around one in 10 people. Depression is fully treatable. It is not a weakness or something that someone can snap out of, and it is not something that lasts forever.

There are many different types of Depression:

- **Clinical depression** is very common but it has no full diagnosis. It means that only a doctor has the power to diagnose you with clinical depression.

- **Depressive episodes** – your doctor may say that you're going through a depressive episode. This is the full name that doctors give depression when they make a diagnosis. They may categorise it as mild, moderate or severe.

- **Recurrent depressive disorder** – if you have a number of depressive episodes, the doctor might say you have a recurrent depressive disorder. Once again, this can be categorised as mild moderate or severe.

- **Reactive depression** – if your doctor thinks that your depression was caused by a stressful event in life, they may say it is reactive.

- **Manic depression** – manic depression is a different illness to depression. This may be known as bipolar disorder. People with this illness have severe highs (mania) and lows (depression).

- **Psychotic depression** – if you are severely depressed, you may start to hallucinate or believe things that aren't true. This is called psychotic.

- **Postnatal depression** – postnatal depression is a common illness which affects 10 to 15 in every hundred women who have a baby. You may get symptoms of those that have other types of depression.

I have even heard that the average age of the first onset of major depression is between 25 and 29 years old.

On the front line to treat depression is medication called antidepressants. This may control some of the symptoms but it usually does little to give sufferers depression-free lives. The drug treatment system has failed.

70 years ago, you were 10 times less likely to suffer from any sort of depression. This clearly shows that the root cause of most depression is not a chemical imbalance as human genes do not change that fast.

Anxiety

Current facts:

- While 2.6% of the UK population experience depression and 4.7% have anxiety problems, as many as 9.7% suffer mixed depression and anxiety, making it the most prevalent mental health problem in the population as a whole.

- Generalised Anxiety Disorder affects between 2–5% of the UK population, yet accounts for as much as 30% of the mental health problems seen by GPs.

- People in their middle years (35 to 59) report the highest levels of anxiety compared to other age groups.

- Four in every ten employed people experience anxiety about their work.

- Fewer than one in ten people have sought help from their GP to deal with anxiety, although those who feel anxious more frequently are much more likely to do this.

- One-fifth of people who have experienced anxiety do nothing to cope with it.

Mental Health Foundation. Retrieved from http://www.mentalhealth.org.uk/help-information/mental-health-statistics/anxiety-statistics/. *Accessed on Nov 2015*

Anxiety is a normal, if unpleasant, part of life, and it can affect us all in different ways and at different times. Whereas stress is something that will come and go as the external factor causing it (be it work, relationship or money problems, etc.) comes and goes, anxiety is something that can persist whether or not the cause is clear to the sufferer.

Anxiety can make a person imagine that things in their life are worse than they really are, and prevent them from confronting their fears. Often, they will think they are going mad, or that some psychological imbalance is at the heart of their woes.

There are many symptoms, both physical and physiological, that happen to individuals when they are anxious:

• a pounding heartbeat

• breathing faster

• palpitations (an irregular heartbeat)

• feeling sick

• chest pains

• headaches

• sweating

• loss of appetite

• feeling faint

• needing the toilet more frequently

• "butterflies" in your tummy

A little anxiety is not bad for you. Everything, as long as it is not chronic, can benefit and strengthen you. When it becomes long-term, illnesses such as hypertension and infections can be contracted.

Current state- Nutritional

Current facts:

- **2 billion people in this world have anaemia, many due to iron deficiency** [1]

- **Vitamin A deficiency (VAD) is the leading cause of preventable blindness in children and increases the risk of disease and death from severe infections** [2]

- **Some of the nutrients, vitamins and minerals needed in everyday life are protein, energy, vitamin A and carotene, vitamin D, vitamin E, vitamin K, thiamine, riboflavin, niacin, vitamin B6, biotin, vitamin B12, folate, vitamin C, antioxidants, calcium, iron, zinc, selenium, magnesium and iodine** [3]

World Health Organisation. Accessed on Nov 2015.

1. http://www.who.int/nutrition/topics/ida/en/

2. http://www.who.int/nutrition/topics/vad/en/

3. http://www.who.int/nutrition/topics/nutrecomm/en/

The current model of nutritional guidelines depicted by the Eat Well plate created in September 2007, states that a third of our daily intake should be starchy carbohydrates, one third of our intake should be fruit and vegetables, and the final third is divided between milk and dairy products, meat and protein and foods high in sugar and fat.

NHS Choices (Nov 2015). The Eat Well Plate. Retrieved from http://www.nhs.uk/Livewell/Goodfood/Pages/eatwell-plate.aspx

This is a rather narrow-minded way of delivering nutritional advice as each individual person and digestive system is different. Some people cannot process carbohydrates as well as others, resulting in excessive body fat storage from an overdose of carbohydrates.

Although the Eat Well plate states that a third of our daily intake should consist of fruit and vegetables, people in society rarely eat 1 to 5 fruit and vegetables per day. It is also not essential for you to have milk or dairy products in your diet.

The quality of the food is a lot different as well. Let's look at ground sources of food first. Soil is now being sprayed with fertilisers and other chemicals to make crops grow quicker and bigger than before. These chemicals have been translated into the food, degrading the quality of the crop. It is a fact that fruit and vegetables have declined in nutrient contents due to the current process of agriculture.

Scientific American (Nov 2015). Dirt Poor: Have Fruits and Vegetables Become Less Nutritious? Retrieved from http://www.scientificamerican.com/article/soil-depletion-and-nutrition-loss/

In addition, these chemicals in the food are foreign to the body and cause other forms of stress for the body as these elements of the food have to be eliminated from the body.

Going up the food chain, the animals we eat are of a poor quality as well. Farming has now been industrialised to the point of factory farms. This is where chickens, fish, lamb, beef, pork and other meat groups are produced in prison like conditions. They are treated as a physical stock and not as living creatures. They are kept within confined spaces, pumped full of steroids, growth hormones and antibiotics so they grow quicker, and fed feed that is unnatural to them as they become fatter and disposed of if unwanted (male chickens are simply thrown away sometimes as they cannot produce eggs). Illness is rife in these settings with many animals dying and rotting in cages. Let me give you an example of how it is. Imagine a hatchback car. The car is designed for 4 people, 5 people maximum. Pack it with 8-15 people. People are on top of each other, squashed and cramped. The only food you get in there is ice cream, chocolate, sugary drinks, sugar covered donuts and an array of sugary carbohydrate foods. You are unable to move; therefore, you cannot burn any calories so the only calories you burn are through breathing.

Someone in the car gets ill, but he is right at the bottom so he can't get out. He dies in the car, infecting people with his smell and illness.

Imagine the stress you would be feeling and taking into your body. Just because they are animals, does not mean they do not feel stress, and this is all translated into the body. We know that stress releases chemicals in the body and if they are constantly there, this can affect the physiology of an individual. It is the same thing with an animal. And when we eat these products, the chemicals and the stresses can be transferred into our system. There have been many occurrences where individuals have changed their diet and felt less stressed, angry and agitated as a result. In some alternative therapies, food is used to treat ADHD and hyperactivity.

Water consumption is also an issue. In essence, we are drinking too little water and some of us are drinking bad quality water which is once again full of foreign agents your body now has to expel.

Most of our diets are very acidic in nature. A mixture of an acidic diet, emotional stress, toxic overload, and/or immune reactions or any process that deprives the cells of oxygen and other nutrients is the perfect place for disease and illness to thrive. It can make it difficult to utilise vital nutrients from food, difficult to produce adequate energy, difficult to repair damaged cells and heavy metal detoxification and can help a tumour to become stronger. A pH of 6.9 can have serious problems and can result in a coma.

Consuming too much animal products (which are acid producing) is one of the main culprits of this imbalance of pH. This coupled with fizzy drinks, coffee and refined grains are damaging us from the inside out. Our bodies are amazing at fighting off any imbalances. Mental and emotional stress, hormone balancing, digestion, physical activity and electromagnetic stress are just some of the tasks your body is doing now to keep you fit and functional. It is always trying to restore optimal health and expel any foreign agents. The optimal way for this to happen , after a period of stress, is to have a period of relaxation. This allows those cells that are working to rebuild and get stronger so it can continue the good fight. The thing is, due to lack of knowledge, individuals are piling on stress to the body at every angle. The body and the cells need adequate energy to keep going which is supplied by nutrition and oxygen; and the downtime to regenerate.

Current state- Chemical

<u>Current facts:</u>

- **Our body can handle and expel up to 1.2 million toxins per day. We are exposed to nearly 2.1 million toxins per day coming from beverages, drugs, parasites, stress, heavy metals, radiation etc.**

Pierce, Cal. (Nov 2015). Receive your Healing and Reclaim Your Health [Book Format]. Retrieved from page 161-162.

We are now, more so than ever, being bombarded with chemicals from a multiple of places.

Starting off with the air we breathe, in urban city environments such as London, when doing research on air pollution, they stated that apart from small areas in the main city centres, the air is "UNLIKELY to cause any adverse health conditions". The word 'unlikely' suggests uncertainty in their sentence. The map literally has only main town centres as high air pollution areas. Adjacent areas are labelled 'safe' even though it only takes seconds to walk from a higher air polluted area to a lower air polluted area. If you have any doubts about this, please type " air pollution in London" on a search engine.

http://www.londonair.org.uk/london/asp/nowcast.asp

Another source of chemicals entering our system is through our water supply. As we all know, our tap water is treated with chemicals making it safe for it to be used by us, the general public. The chemicals used are something called 'solution' to make particles bigger to be removed and chlorine. The statement on Thames Water website is as follows: "we turn raw water into safe and wholesome water".

http://www.thameswater.co.uk/cycles/accessible/water_cycle.html

Let me ask you a question, would you take a raw vegetable, wash it in chemicals to make it 'safe' and then consume it? It doesn't make sense.

That is a very strange choice of words from one of the biggest suppliers of tap water, that's all I'm saying.

Plastic contamination was also a big issue. There was an epidemic due to certain plastics that were given to the general public due to its disruptive nature within the body. The three that were under scrutiny were PVC (polyvinyl chloride), PS (polystyrene) and PC (polycarbonate). These are commonly found in children's toys, shower curtains, wallpaper, BPA and Styrofoam. These plastics were found to have hormone disrupters, reproductive organ disrupters, cancers and a variety of other health problems.

KEY POINTS TO TAKE FROM ABOVE

- Our society is experiencing very serious health problems

- UK statistic- one in four people this year will experience a mental health issue

- UK statistic- less than one in two people will contract cancer

- The Eat Well plate model, brought in the UK in 2007, is a very narrow-minded view on nutrition as it states a 'one size fits all' attitude to nutrition

- Less than half the population is consuming 5 pieces of fruit and vegetables a day.

- The quality of the soil that grows our food is worse as it is full of pesticides

- Animal products are not being reared properly

- We are moving less

- Our body movement is affecting our posture

- We need to reclaim our health back

- Air pollution is considered 'unlikely' to harm us

- Only 4 pollutants are measured on the air pollution scale- Nowcast

- Plastics can be very disruptive for the body

- Water supply- they cleanse raw water into safe and wholesome water apparently

Now, we are a constantly evolving organism with millions of reactions going on in our bodies at every second. This means we are constantly changing. Now, this change can be for the better or for the worse, depending on how we treat our body/mind/spirit. It is never too late to start making changes in our diet and lifestyle to swing the favour back towards health and vitality. We have, as a society, over complicated what we need to do in order to achieve that. We have multiple companies claiming with artificial means to help us obtain health. The problem is, these solutions given to us are classified as foreign agents to our bodies. Medicine, drugs and pills have only come around within the last 150 years or so, yet our bodies have been around for approximately 200,000 years as sapiens. So much advancement, with new drugs being created and approved frequently, is creating another stress in our body.

Let us take health back the Natural Way. There is a saying 'Let thy food be thy medicine and let thy medicine be thy food'. Funnily enough, this is the statement that was said by the founder of medicine, Hippocrates.

We need to re-educate ourselves about our health. We have so much to learn as a community of people. We have been told or sold things that may not serve us well or have no real benefit to our lives.

We are now at an evolutionary period in our time. It is the period of change. We have to take back the power of education and relearn who we really are. Start with your health now. Get to know your mind, your body and your spirit. There is a vast amount of power within you.

Live the Stress-Less Way of Life.

My Story - How Stress-Less was born

The journey of the birth of Stress-Less was not a straight-forward journey, but then, no great story is. It started with a young child with a fascination of the mind.

The study of the mind, decision making and psychology has been of great interest to me. How do people rationalise the decisions they make? What is good and what is bad? Is there ever really a universal good or bad or is it all subjective?

For example, if someone steals, does that make them a bad person? If he is stealing to provide for his family, are his actions justified? If he is a product of his environment, is he solely accountable?

These questions going through a 14-year old's mind is not normal. Yet, they were going through my mind. Growing up in urban London, you can sometimes feel like the odds are stacked up against you. You see many people fall into the trap of crime and negativity. Being constantly surrounded by this style of living can influence you and can build a rational case for committing such acts. "If everyone is doing it and everyone is getting away with it, why can't I?" No one wants to be the only one without and you can feel like that sometimes.

What you find is that individuals have trouble with convictions of plans. Everyone has dreams and goals coming from different areas in their lives e.g. career, love, finances, friendships etc. This is a basic human characteristic. Whether we are talking about people in upper class circles or people below the line of poverty. It is universal.

The two main reasons we don't go on to fulfill these goals are because we become impatient and scared. Impatience doesn't trust the process of learning and developing. It is this phase of achieving that turns you into a master of your chosen field, and this applies to all areas. Let's take for example money. About 70% of people who win the lottery on average go broke or file for bankruptcy. Now, if we were told that we would receive millions of pounds for doing nothing, I'm sure we could come up with a list of things that we would do and get, and none of us would say we would ever go bankrupt.

If the journey of achieving your dream or goal is not included, the lessons that would need to be learnt will not be included, making failure more likely. You have little appreciation of what you get fast.

The second which is fear is more prominent in our society today. The fear of taking that step into the unknown is one of the primary reasons for why people don't chase their dreams. Anything unknown is seen as scary. Once we are in our comfort zone, where everything is familiar and almost automated, it is difficult to push yourself out and take that step. On top of that, we create limiting beliefs about our abilities so we rationalise it and say it's 'safer' to stay in your known zone. Our life can become stagnant and unfulfilling. We dread the weekdays and look forward so much to the weekend. We try so hard to forget about our lives and enjoy ourselves. Often using stimulants e.g. alcohol to take us into a state of self-hypnosis. Our body takes most of the abuse when it comes to the pursuit of happiness and fulfillment.

This is why at Stress-Less, developing someone's mind is at the forefront of what we want to achieve with our clients. To create that mind-set change is fundamental to success in all endeavours in life. Whether we have emotional issues, limiting beliefs, weak mind-set, lack of persistence or drive, or negative outlook, these traits are not fixed. They can be changed, developed and removed to only have things that serve your desired outcome.

As stated before, once your mind-set isn't healthy, it normally has repercussions on other aspects of your health. You start to eat and drink unhealthy products, chemical imbalances form in the body and effective physical movement is limited. When the body becomes out of sync with its natural processes, illnesses and diseases form more easily and rapidly. Diseases like cancers, auto immune diseases, high blood pressure, diabetes, obesity, posture problems, aches and pains formation and mental illness are all more common now compared to years ago. The only thing that we can correlate to this rise in disease is that our lifestyle has greatly changed. Genes and other molecular factors have now been accused for our health problems but this is deferring from the truth. We are not taking care of ourselves as much as we should.

Society conditioning tells us that you need to eat this for this and eat that for that. We have to have stimulants to feel free and forget all your worries. The News tells us that there is a lot of negativity in the world, that we are all alone in a crazy world and you have to fend for yourself and yourself alone.

We have become a society that is more worried about profit than helping others. Major companies are taking shortcuts in order to drive down their prices, which in turn drives down the quality of the products. This is relevant in the agricultural and farming industries. There are so many toxins being pumped into the air changing the O-zone layer.

Stress-Less' mission is to create real change. Bringing a culture of wellness and helping one another. We are all on this journey of life together trying to fulfill our dreams and goals. Trying to experience that natural bliss, that feeling of natural ecstasy, feeling alive.

We are constantly looking for the next thing that is going to make us healthy, to cure all our ailments so we can live a healthy life. We are always looking for that thing that when we get it, we will feel, look, and act happy and healthy. Isn't that what everyone wants? The problem with this is that it leaves you open to external sources telling you what you need. You are the best nutritionist and doctor for yourself. Take control of your health and your life. Start a preventive focused approach to your health, rather than only reacting when you feel dis-ease. Give yourself back the power of health. Feeding your mind, body and spirit with what it is calling for is the best and most natural way of bliss as it is ever lasting without any side effects.

The Stress-Less Way of Life model

There is hope.

Taking charge of your health is the first step to having a happier and healthier life. As stated before, our body is a constantly evolving organism that is capable of change. Cells are dying and being reborn every second. What you do now will affect how your cells grow in the future. This means starting to make changes now will change how your cells will evolve in the future. You can rebuild yourself and your health cell by cell.

The one thing that affects the cell development is the stress on the body and cells. When I say stress, I am talking about physiological stress. All the stresses in our lives are interpreted in the body as physiological stress, whether it is created by our mind, our food or other factors.

Stress is not bad. Let's get that illusion destroyed now. Stress helps us to survive. When our ancestors were living off the land, stress was a key to getting away from danger.

The problem with stress these days is that it is turning chronic. The wonderful ability of the human mind is that we make our thoughts real. Now this allows us to manifest ideas or dreams into creation. This is how some of the greatest inventions have been created and some of the greatest minds have been formulated. On the flip side, it can also show our doubts, fears and insecurities as if they are real. This is the thing that limits us. This in turn creates stress in the body due to the lack of fulfillment.

When we create stress merely through thought alone, it results in the capability to create constant stress in the body. In addition to this, the different stresses that come within our lives can easily turn into chronic stress.

We have to create a balance of stress within our body, increasing it where it needs to be increased and decrease likewise. This is the only way to stay fit, sharp and healthy.

The different types of stress that the body experiences are:

1. **Physical Stress**- exercise is a primary form of physical stress to the body. Exercise can be both good and bad for our bodies. A good form is when' your body develops, gets stronger in the required areas and you maintain a good level of energy. A bad form of stress through exercise is over-exercising. This is when your body is over-stimulated through exercise, causing too much stress on the body, actually having an adverse effect and making your body weaker.

2. **Nutritional stress**- anything we put in our mouth affects our nutritional stress. A good form of nutritional stress is when you eat the right amount of macronutrients for your dietary type; drink plenty of water, along with eating fruits and vegetables. A bad form of nutritional stress is when you eat junk food, drink fizzy drinks and have an intake of ingredients high in sugar.

3. **Mental stress**- as stated earlier, the mind has the power to influence the body. Emotions are therefore a form of mental stress. A positive form is a happy emotion e.g. happiness and joy. A negative form is an emotion of fear, doubt, anger and feeling unfulfilled.

4. **Body Temperature stress**- your body should maintain a temperature of around 37 degrees. Over or under this level of temperature can cause stress to our bodies.

5. **Electromagnetic stress**- this is the wave signals we receive in our atmosphere. Even though they are unseen and there is not a lot we can do about it, we need to be aware that there is this form of stress affecting our body. A good form of electromagnetic stress is from natural sunlight. It is classified a good source of vitamin D. A bad form of electromagnetic stress is microwave signals and signals emitted of electrical appliances.

6. **Chemical stress**- these forms of stress can be from within the body or foreign agents ingested into the body. The end result is that your body will either be boosted by them or have to find a way to

eliminate them. A good form of stress is your hormones that are naturally released in your body. For example, serotonin is a good hormone for the brain. A bad form of stress is hormone disrupters found in some plastics.

Another important part of maintaining a healthy lifestyle is balancing out the 'stress' response with the 'rest and repair' response in the body. This is the most important part of the stress response. Failure to enter this zone results in chronic stress, fatigue, illness, disease and can cause death.

Some forms of good stress set off this rest and repair response in the body, but not all of them do. The best time for the rest and repair response is when you are in a relaxed state.

Forms of relaxed state:

1. **Sleep**- sleep is essential to our body's development. This is the time when the growth hormone is released and you go through two stages of regeneration in sleep – physical which is a regeneration of the cells and physiological regeneration which is the regeneration of hormones, energy levels etc.

2. **Meditation**- meditation is sometimes known as conscious sleeping. There are many forms of meditation but the key principle is taking your mind away from the cycles of thinking and moving it to a place where it's more relaxed. The two main categories of meditation are contemplation meditation and concentration meditation.

3. **Massage**- this is a form of rejuvenating the body and the muscles with pressure applied. This is to relieve tension and imbalances in the body. Once again, there are many forms of massage e.g. Sports massage, acupressure, deep tissue and seated chair massage.

With creating the favourable stress balance of more good stress than bad, and more time in rest and repair, the body will start to feel and work better. You will increase your energy levels and your health will improve. You will start to think differently about situations. Things will start to click into place and start to make sense.

Start to live the Stress-Less Life.

The Stress-Less Principle- Our Philosophy

The Stress-Less way of life has one governing principle that we live by, the G.A.I.N.E.D principle. It is something that if you apply to every area of your life, you will evolve, grow and be successful. It can be used for your health, career, relationships, family, finances etc. If you don't follow this principle, it will become very difficult to track any achievements. With this comes complacency, a lack of motivation and worse of all, settling for mediocre. This thought should be running through your mind with every situation you take.

This is the G.A.I.N.E.D way of thinking.

The **G.A.I.N.E.D** way of thinking is built on the principle that you can achieve anything you put your time and energy into. The acronym stands for:

G- Gradual

A- And

I- Intentional

N- Never

E- Ending

D- Development

Gradual And Intentional Never Ending Development means that anything you want to achieve, whether it be good health, more money, more vitality, better relationships, to be less dependent on stimulants or for more mental clarity, you need to invest time and effort. Let the stories of countless successful individuals: Bill Gates' first business failed, Jim Carrey used to be homeless, Richard Branson was labelled dyslexic and Steven King's first novel was rejected 30 times. All these individuals did not allow setbacks to hold them back from learning and developing their lives. Their processes of success didn't happen overnight, there is a process, an art in the journey where they effectively developed themselves for their success. As it is said, there is beauty in the struggle. You need to entrench the G.A.I.N.E.D principle into everything you do and you will never go wrong.

How to apply G.A.I.N.E.D into your life

With areas that you wish to improve, dedicate time and energy to these endeavours. Study them, or find an expert in the fields and seek advice. Create a plan. List where you are and where you want to be. Write down steps on how to get to the next level. Track your progress at the end of each day and ask yourself 'what can I do tomorrow to get closer to my goal?'

Task- How Much Time Have You Really Got?

Instructions

1. Draw a graph with the X axis being 'Hours' going to 24 and the Y axis being 'Years' going to 70.

2. On the Years axis, mark a line on how many years you have been alive

On the hours per day axis:

3. On the hours per day axis, mark off how many hours you sleep per night

4. Mark off how much time you spend commuting per day

5. Mark off how much time you have at work/school

6. Mark off how many hours you spend in a state of distraction per day e.g. watching television, listening to music, casually browsing the internet

7. Mark off how much time you spend eating per day

After you see how much time you actually have to spend on yourself and improvement, you may be surprised about the time you actually have left. Remember, this is based on the presence that you have a happy and healthy life up to the age of 70, which a lot of people do not reach due to illness. Cherish the time you have and invest in yourself and your wealth.

Questionnaires

I have devised a series of questions for you to answer in order for you to get an indication of where you are currently. This can help you differentiate the areas of high concern that need to be tackled immediately and other areas that are not such a high priority. They are divided into the types of stress our bodies' experience. I use this questionnaire with all my clients so a plan can be devised about the best outcome. Fill it in and see your score.

Physical Body

1. How often do you use a microwave oven?

2. Do you have mercury amalgam fillings in your mouth?

3. Do you have two different kinds of metal in your mouth i.e. gold/silver/mercury amalgam?

4. How often do you use artificial sweeteners?

5. Do you find that you often burp after meals or get gas?

6. Do you eat canned fish more frequently than fresh fish?

7. Do you commonly eat meat (beef, chicken, turkey) from sources other than a free range or hormone free source?

8. Do you drink tap water?

9. Do you have difficulty burning fat around the belly, hips or thighs even with exercise?

10. Do you have an excessive appetite and/or sweet cravings?

11. Do you experience adnominal pain, cramps or discomfort more than twice a week?

12. Do you live in the same time zone you were born in?

13. Do you travel across time zones more than once a month?

14. How often do you wake up feeling un-rested and in need of more sleep?

15. How often do you wake up at night between 1:00am and 4:00am, and have a hard time falling back to sleep?

16. Do you do shift work that requires you to stay up at night?

17. How often do you typically go more than 4 hours without eating?

18. Have you tried diets to lose weight?

19. Do you eat your largest meal in the evening?

20. How often do you experience constipation or stools that are compact or hard to pass?

20 questions

Mental Body

1. Do you worry over job, income or money problems?

2. Do you feel isolated or lonely?

3. Have you had reduced contact with friends (feeling antisocial) or an increase in contact because you feel you need to vent your frustrations or stresses on others?

4. Do you have any sort of medication prescribed by a doctor due to stress or a psychological disorder?

5. Do you feel your sex drive is lower than normal for you?

6. Do you commonly lose more than two days a year due to illness?

7. Would you consider your life to be out of balance in terms of stress?

8. Do you feel you have an overactive mind?

9. When you have a bad experience, do you repeatedly think about it?

10. Do you have more negative thoughts or feelings than positive ones?

11. Do you often feel anxious?

12. Do you feel stressed due to a lack of intimacy in one or more relationships?

13. Are any of your relationships causing you stress?

14. Do you often get upset when things go wrong?

15. Do you lash out at others?

16. Do you experience mood swings?

17. Do you feel like you are out of control of your feelings and emotions?

18. Are you currently unhappy with your main activity of the day? (Work, parent, student etc.)

19. Do you believe that children are built with an inherited talent that is fixed and nearly impossible to develop?

20. Do you use recreational drugs?

21. Do you truly feel like you are incapable of achieving your dreams?

22. Are you lacking in developing your mental ability?

22 questions

Nutritional Body

1. Do you shop for food less frequently than every four days?

2. Do you eat more packaged (frozen or canned) fruit and vegetables than fresh?

3. Do you eat more cooked vegetables than raw?

4. Do you buy more non-organic vegetables than organic vegetables?

5. Do you eat vegetables with fewer than two meals per day?

6. Do you typically eat store-bought eggs from caged raised chickens (as opposed to free range eggs)?

7. How often do you eat from fast food restaurants?

8. Do you eat TV dinners, or highly processed foods more than three times a week?

9. How often do you eat snacks from vending machines?

10. Do you eat white bread more often than whole grain breads?

11. Do you eat quick cooked grains more often than slow cooked organic whole grains?

12. How often do you use white sugar as a sweetener?

13. Do you often get hungry or crave sweets within two hours of eating?

14. Do you consume more than 3 drinks a day containing caffeine or sugar?

15. Do you consume fat whilst eating?

16. Do you consume pasteurised, homogenised milk/cheese or non-organic yogurt often (3 times a week or more)?

17. Do you eat non-organic red meat more than once every 4 days?

18. Do you consume products containing hydrogenated oils?

19. Do you eat nuts or seeds that are roasted or salted?

20. Do you use standard white table salt?

21. Do you eat some form of store-bought desserts such as ice cream, cookies, donuts, cakes and pies frequently (3+ times a week)?

22. Do you often skip breakfast?

23. Do you frequently skip meals?

24. Do you tend to have a hard time staying awake after lunch?

25. Do you find that regardless of how much you eat you get hungry quickly?

26. Do you eat more or less when stressed than when not stressed?

26 questions

The Results

Physical Body Results

Foreign Agents

Q1-6- If you answered yes **to 2 or more questions**, read Foreign Agents section on page 44

Chemical Imbalance

Q7-11- If you answered yes **to 2 or more questions**, read Chemical Imbalance on page 44

Sleep

Q12-16- If you answered yes **to 2 or more questions**, read Sleep on page 45

Bad habits, Poor Body

Q17-20- If you answered yes **to 2 or more questions s**, read Bad Habits, Poor Body on page 46

Mental Body Results

Rewire the Brain

Q1-6- If you answered yes **to 3 or more questions**, Read Rewire the Brain on page 47

Metacognition

Q7-11- If you answered yes **to 2 or more questions**, read Metacognition on page 47

Emotional Intelligence

Q12-17- If you answered yes **to 2 or more questions**, read Emotional Intelligence on page 47

Mind-set Training and Mastery

Q18-22- If you answered yes **to 2 or more questions**, read Mind-set Training and Mastery on page 48

<u>Nutritional Body Results</u>

Food freshness

Q1-9 - If you answered yes **to 4 or more questions**, read Food freshness on page 49

Refined carbohydrate over intake

Q10-15- If you answered yes **to 2 or more questions,** read refined carbohydrates over intake on page 49

Quality of food

Q16-21 - If you answered yes **to 2 or more questions**, read Quality of Food on page 50

You are when you eat

Q22-26 - If you answered yes **to 2 or more questions**, read You Are When You Eat on page 51

Recommendations

After going through your results and finding out your areas of weakness, here is a list of recommendations that you should incorporate into your life in order to create more balance in your life. Start with the biggest priority and work your way through.

Physical

Foreign Agents

- **Watch out for electromagnetic waves**- you may be overexposed to radiation by extremely low frequencies (ELF) by electronic devices e.g. Computers, mobile phones, microwaves, electric motors and TV's.

- **Watch out for the contaminations in society**- metal and plastic contaminations are overlooked, yet very real in our society. In an effort to cut costs, companies are using poor quality materials to store food. When heated, these can transfer into our food. In terms of metal, canned goods can be stored in their metal casing for years on end. As time goes on, some of the properties from the metal can transfer into the liquid. Store food in glass or ceramics. Eat as many fresh ingredients as possible e.g. instead of canned tuna, buy fresh tuna.

- **Watch out for hidden chemicals**- a lot of preservatives have been added to our food in the pursuit of extending the shelf life of products. Most of the ingredients we do not know and have never heard of; some we can't even pronounce. Most of these ingredients are foreign to the body and the body treats it like it is under attack. Limit the amount of processed foods in your diet and eat as much fresh food as possible.

Chemical Imbalances

To start to balance out the chemicals in your body:

- **Calliper testing**- skin fold testing in certain areas can indicate an excess hormone in the body. From then, we can design a plan of action to help to balance out your body. Enquire about calliper testing through Stress-Less at our studio situated in London.

- **Eat more dark green vegetables**- these have a tremendous quality of detoxing and neutralising the body. Vegetables such as broccoli, spinach, kale, cucumber etc. (organic where possible)

- **Drink more water**- this can help flush the body of toxins

- **Relax**-the 'rest and repair' response in the body allows your cells to rebuild and grow back stronger.

Sleep

Top tips to improve your sleep:

- **Turn off your Wi-Fi and your telephone signal 30 minutes before sleep**-electromagnetic waves can affect your internal chemistry making it difficult for you to get a full and proper night's sleep.

- **Make it to bed by 10.30pm latest**- our physiological and physical regeneration phases start generally at around 10.30pm. If you sleep at this time, you will receive the maximum amount of cellular and mental regeneration.

- **Use natural light-** our brains interpret light as daytime and darkness at night time. If we have artificial light in our house e.g. House lights, our brain can be tricked into thinking it is still daytime. Our brain requires around 2-3 hours to shut down and become rested. Instead of having lights in the house, open the curtains and use the sun light to light your house.

- **Have a relaxing bath 30-60 minutes before bed**- having a bath with magnesium flakes included is a great way to relax the body. Magnesium is the mineral associated with relaxation in the body so adding the flakes can help to relax the body and the mind.

- **Do not have a big meal after 6.30pm**- the body takes around 4 hours to process big cooked meals. If you are to eat after this time, a raw salad that consists of 75% of your meal is advised.

Bad habits, Poor Body

Top tips for bad habits, poor body:

- **Have a meal or a snack every 2-3 hours where possible**- by having a meal every 2-3 hours, you maintain a healthy blood sugar level and don't overburden the hormone insulin. Insulin is the key hormone associated with type 2 diabetes and excess weight around the mid-section.

- **Break up your meals appropriately**- you would want your biggest meal to be breakfast. Reason being is that your body will have the adequate amount of time to break down and utilise the food taken in. Lunch is the next big meal, but smaller than breakfast and dinner is the smallest meal. Your portion of meals should look like a downwards triangle, biggest at the top, smallest at the bottom.

- **Do not diet**- diets are designed to make you lose weight, but it is not helping you lose the required weight: body fat. The problem with most diets is that they make you lose muscle (which weighs more than body fat) making you look like you have lost a huge amount of weight. Also, when you return to your normal eating, your metabolism hasn't adjusted and your body still thinks it's going through a famine (that's what a diet does to your body). As it's still in famine mode, any food consumed will be stored for utilisation at a later date when the famine returns. You therefore end up putting on more weight than before. Create lifestyle changes that will help you achieve a healthy weight in a safe way. Look at getting a Stress-Less Meal Plan created for you.

- **Detox the body-** through the years, our bodies accumulates waste products which have to be dispose of by the liver. The liver can be over burdened with work due to the nature of our body's elimination process. There is a very simple way we can aid the liver and our body in this elimination process: by drinking a litre of water every morning before we consume anything. This starts the movement of waste through the system and is also a great way to start to flush it out.

Mental

Rewire the brain

- **Your life is powered 90% by your subconscious mind**- tapping into your subconscious mind and recognising what tapes are running in there could be the most important thing you do to manage your mental state. The 'Rewire the Brain' course helps you to understand the meaning behind the subconscious mind, and how to break it down so that it is no longer inhibiting your progress mentally and physically.

Metacognition

- **Start to examine at your thoughts**- your thoughts shape your outlook in life. It shapes what is drawn towards you, away from you, what you say, do and achieve. It is the foundation block of building a strong mind and a strong body. Letting them run loose with any regulation is like letting a wild animal out in a crowded zoo. People will be hurt. Start to look at what thoughts run through your mind and whether they are serving you well.

- **Take the Metacognition course**- if you are new to the observation of your thoughts, take the Metacognition course and it will give you a more detailed procedure on how to start doing this. Contact the Stress-Less Team for more information.

Emotional Intelligence

- **Learn about emotional intelligence**- emotional states, when acted upon with no contemplation, stops us from saying or acting how we would want to act in a desired manner. It can affect relationships and the results we get out of our endeavours. Being in control of our state of mind is therefore critical to success and achieving objectives. Take the emotional intelligence course to control and develop your emotional strength and skills. Contact the Stress-Less Team for more information.

Mind-set training and Mastery

- **Have a plan**- one of the key reasons to why our mind-sets are not directed towards successful pursuits is because we don't know what we want or we don't know how to get to where we want in a strategic and formulated way. Find out where you currently are, what your ideal situation is, and create methodical steps to reaching your goal.

- **Find out who you are**- we are bombarded in the media of celebrities and public figures that we are supposed to emulate. We spend the majority of our life playing catch up, forgetting who we are and chasing an image of who we think or who the world wants us to be. Take away the titles that have been given to you and ask yourself 'who are you? What is the essence of you?' From working this out, you will have a better idea of yourself.

- **Take the Mind-set training and mastery course**- we have given you a structured way of developing your mind-set towards success and mastery on our course. Take the course and develop your mind-set towards your true goals in life. Contact the Stress-Less Team for more information.

Nutrition

Food freshness

- **Fresh is best**- When shopping for food, buy fresh food once every 4 days. This is the best way to ensure your food has a good amount of nutrients within them. After this, food can lose nutrient content.

- **Try to go to a butchers or a fishmonger for your meat and fish-** Ask if their produce is free range. The best source is free range and organic. Just organic means that the animals still could have been served food which is not natural in their diet for growth acceleration purposes. Check to see where the fish came from. Stay away from fish farms, they are similar to caged chickens in a factory farm.

- **Buy fresh produce from whole food shops**- there is a lot of great produce in whole food shops. They do not have your general off-the-mill products found in your supermarket. They have a claim of being eco-friendly and having less toxic chemicals in their food. Just be wary about the food you buy.

- **Source your local farmer's market**- farmer's markets are a great way to get local produce. All produce are grown in the UK and have an eco-friendly approach to food, most of them say their produce is organic or bio-dynamic.

Refined carbohydrates intake

- **Use natural sweeteners**- refined and artificial sweeteners have too many chemicals and bleach added that destroy the quality of the food. White refined sugar is one of the worst forms of refined sweeteners and is known to have the same effects on the brain as cocaine. Stick to natural sweeteners like raw honey, lemon or natural sweeteners such as stevia.

- **Avoid sugary products**- items with too much sugar can be very corrosive for your internal system. Sugar is very acidic by nature. Often in foods, they do not put 'sugar' on the label, they mask it as fructose/sucrose/glucose or corn syrup (which is cheaper to make and a lot worse than refined sugar). Look at the labelling of your food and see if any of these names are there. For your best bet, stick to natural raw ingredients. You can now download a sugar content scanner app telling you how much sugar is in each product you buy.

Quality of food

- **Buy the best produce**- quality should come before anything. Sometimes we look after physical things more than our own internal system. We would not fill a car with the wrong oil so let's start to fill our body with the things it needs. You are investing in yourself. Good quality produce has a higher quantity of nutrients within them so after a high quality meal, you feel more nourished often with eating less. Organic, free range, free from chemicals and ethically farmed products are the best forms of quality foods.

- **Avoid unhealthy food sources**- these foods are often filled with 'empty calories'. Empty calories are ones which have no nutritional value to your body but still fill you with calories. The result is that you end up feeling hungry soon after your meal as your reason for eating (to receive nourishment) has not been fulfilled.

- **Don't be fooled by so-called health benefits**- companies are becoming very smart with the wording of some of their products and packaging. They are using certain words and phrases that indicate health when really there is very little change in the product itself. This is often done with little regulation on what can and what cannot be displayed on a product. You will be surprised about what companies can get away with. Watch out for these statements on food products by these companies. If they say they are 'reduced fat', how much by and what type of fat? Investigate what you are eating and don't be fooled by the language they use.

You are when you eat

- **Timings of meals**- there has been many options about timing of meals. As a general rule, breakfast should be within one hour of waking, lunch should be mid-day and dinner should be around six o'clock. This is not the case for everyone as people have different work schedules and lifestyles. As a general rule, the best time to eat is when your body is calling for nourishment. Always start your day with water (preferably with room temperature water with lemon included). The best thing to do is to listen to the body and give it what it needs. You should definitely have your main meals at the beginning and middle of the day, and light meals in the evening with supplements of food in-between if needed.

- **Quantities of meals**- by a general rule of thumb, breakfast should be your biggest meal of the day. This should set your day off correctly and keep you on track mentally and physically. This also correlates to the amount of energy you need for bodily functions (hormone release and waste removal). Lunch is your second biggest, giving you that push you need to keep going during the day at your main day's activity. In the evening, your body is going into the rest and repair phase so a big meal is unnecessary. Just something light to supplement your body with nutrients ready for bed.

- **Ideal macronutrient percentages**- this is what normally goes wrong with weight gain and weight loss. Individuals are commonly eating the wrong amount of the macronutrients so they are putting on weight even though they are eating correctly. Download the macronutrient assessment questionnaire to find out what predisposition you have for each macronutrient group and how much you should eat of each.

- **When not to eat**- eating at the wrong time can affect how well your body can utilise the food and digest into the system. The first rule is if you eat a heavy meal late in the evening, you are more likely to put on weight as your body has no way of utilising the energy given from the food. There is also a list of do's and don'ts with when not to eat and the psychological reasons of why we cannot lose weight. Download the 'When not to eat' course to work through different issues you may have. Contact the Stress-Less Team for more information.

Start your new life now

The Stress-Less way of life is exactly that, a way of life. It is not a quick fix pill, a special diet or a new exercise that will give you amazing results in days. It takes consistency, dedication and willpower. We often struggle with these things when it comes to health, so let's relate it to something universal. In a workplace environment, in order to get to the top, you have to work hard, pass the tests and strive for greatness, otherwise, you will fall short of what it takes. We all invest our time and our money in the goal of financial freedom, to live a life where we can do what we love, when we want. So let's transfer that energy into our health. In order to become truly healthy, we need to work hard and learn and study about our minds and our bodies. We have to preserve our one most precious asset, our body. This is what gives us the time and the energy to pursue our dreams, to be able to fulfill the people we are truly supposed to be. It is time we invest into our health. This brings the best return, physical, mental and nutritional liberation. Join the Stress-Less movement and live the fullest life you can ever imagine.

www.ingramcontent.com/pod-product-compliance
Lightning Source LLC
Chambersburg PA
CBHW071254280526
45788CB00004B/1711